Preface

I was "this close"......*this close,* to [obscured by barcode] had had one

more earache. They were a consta[obscured] kid. Back in the day,

and I'm aging myself here, you'd put [obscured] ps in your ears while your mom

would shove cotton balls in them. The ear drops supposedly helped the aching go

away.

Honestly, I don't remember. To think about the treatment now is just ridiculous.

Ear drops to fix an ear ache? Really? Today, you give a kid an antibiotic and a

revisit in two weeks.

Maybe that's why my ear aches kept reoccurring. Maybe that's why we ran out of

cotton balls in our house when my mom wanted to remove her nail polish and

started dropping the F bomb that there weren't any cotton balls and then looked

at me like I had a pork chop around my neck.

But, as the god's were watching over me, I didn't have to have my tonsils

removed. It was considered major surgery having your tonsils taken out back in

the 1970's, and I was definitely looking forward to getting some ice cream with a

few nurses to fluff my pillows and get my first experience at staying in a hospital.

No dice.

Sometimes I almost wished it had happened. If it had happened, maybe I wouldn't be where I am today. Where am I today?

Where I am today is dizzy. I'm dizzy. I'm sick. I'm tired. I also want to wear a helmet 24 hours a day even if I'm at home. The helmet is not to keep my three German Shepherds from licking my face, or to protect myself from Google street cameras exposing my fake identity (or identify me as picking my underwear out of my butt, or providing sign language to a guy who almost ran me over).

No.

The helmet is for my own protection and for the protection of my walls, and priceless pieces of art from Target.

I have drop attacks which is the severest form of Meniere's disease.

I have migraines with headaches.

I have bi-lateral Meniere's Disease.

I am a bi-lateral cochlear recipient and am naturally deaf without them.

What is Meniere's Disease?

To gain a little perspective, and to see if you may be one of those who has Meniere's Disease, please let me explain the history behind it and what it is. Meniere's disease is a disorder of the inner ear which causes episodes of vertigo, ringing in the ears (tinnitus), a feeling of fullness or pressure in the ear, and fluctuating hearing loss. In other words, you pretty much feel like total shit on the endless spinning wheel at a kid's playground while having a constant buzzing from what you would think were bees trying to build a hive in your ear canal.

A typical attack of Meniere's disease is preceded by a fullness in one ear. Hearing fluctuation or changes in tinnitus may also precede an attack. And by the word, "attack," I don't mean dropping you down like the kind of attacks you see on the six o'clock news. Meniere's is sneaky like a politician. It decides to show up whenever it wants, doesn't support your issues by making you feel better and It's constantly a pain in my ass.

 A Meniere's episode generally involves severe vertigo, or spinning, imbalance, nausea and vomiting. The average attack lasts anywhere from two to four hours.

3

Following an attack, most people, like myself, find that they are exhausted and must sleep for several hours. Most people at my age would love to take naps during any time of the day. However, if there is any sort of spinning or vomiting on oneself involved, keep me out of it. Wait. I'm in it. I'm totally in it. I'm actually forced to take nap time with my blankey and I wasn't even offered cookies and juice afterward.

There is a large amount of variability in the duration of symptoms. Some people experience brief "shocks," and others have constant unsteadiness. During attacks, the eyes jump around, or in the most severe cases, people have drop attacks like me. This isn't an endorsement for any type of award. Drop attacks are not fun. It's like having invisible demons throw you across the room. Think, "Exorcist." It just happens. There is no walking up the stairs backwards and vomiting green slime. That's just for the movies. I didn't pee on any priceless Persian carpets either. You just feel like you're falling or spinning and falling or being thrown. You black out. You can severely injure yourself. You can kill yourself. *(dramatic music starts....)*

Meniere's episodes may occur in clusters, that is, several attacks may occur within a short period of time. However, years may pass between episodes. This is my case, and I'll explain a little bit about that later.

Meniere's affects 0.2% of the population. It usually starts confined to one ear (for me, it started in my right ear), but it often extends to involve both ears over time (my left ear was affected one year later). In most cases of Meniere's, a progressive hearing loss occurs in the affected ear(s).

What Damage is Done By Meniere's Disease?

Hair cell death. No, not the hair on your head. Truth be told, I have more hair on my head to provide fake hair for at least 10,000 Barbie dolls. My mother used to complain about combing my hair when I was a little girl because she couldn't get a wire brush thru it. Really? As a seven year old little girl, did you sit there like Marcia Brady constantly combing your hair while admiring yourself in the mirror? I didn't. My mother had a hard time getting me into the bathtub to wash the dirt from underneath my fingernails let alone comb my thick mane of hair that spanned the entire length of my backside. Believe it or not, you do have hair cells in the inner ear. Cochlear (hearing) cells are the most sensitive. The death of hair cells causes a reduction in hearing, or progression of hearing loss. The other issue is mechanical disruptions to the inner ear. This causes chronic unsteadiness, when people are not having attacks.

How Common is Meniere's Disease?

Basically, you can equate Meniere's to be as common as multiple sclerosis. 200 out of 100,000 people get the disease. Most are over 40 years old and there is no exclusivity between genders. Currently, there is no cure which really pisses me off because I've been dealing with this disease since I've been 21 years old. Let's just say that patience is not a virtue of mine.

I laugh at myself because I'm 49 and have had all of this heartily handed to me by the Big Guy upstairs.

This book is about coping with Meniere's Disease. What the disease is really about, and what are the symptoms. This book is also about migraines, drop attacks, medications, psychological and physical side effects and the toll it takes on you and your family.

I was called a liability at one time. I was called a piece of shit by a woman because I didn't understand sign language, thus she didn't believe I couldn't hear her. I've been dismissed or passed over in conversations because I just didn't understand what people were saying.

This book is for people who suffer like me with Meniere's Disease and all the great stuff that comes with it. I want to tell you my story, and thru my story I want to share with you:

- Coping mechanisms

- Using your other senses to make up for the one you lost

- Dealing with the dizziness and how to pass the time

- Overcoming depression and isolation

- Having a backup plan for emergencies

- Things, places and people to avoid

- Embrace being imperfect because being perfect is just plain boring

- Expectations from others

- Medications and resources

I'm not a serious person. As you can see by my writing, I look at my condition with a sense of humor. At times, I want to throw something against the wall for all of the problems it has caused me, but if I have to live with this, I might as well poke some fun at myself and the situation God has provided me or otherwise it would drive me insane.

I've been called insane, you know. Just giving you a heads up on that one.

I Can Finally Hear Birds:

A Candid, Comical And Intimate Journey About Hearing Loss,

Meniere's Disease And Cochlear Implants

By Nancy Chovancek

Dedication

To my husband, Dave. Thank you for being there for me to lean on, fall into, pass out on and use as a wall.

You are my rock.

Chapter 1 - The Drop

"You blacked out." Dave looked over me as he spoke those first words.

I laid on the hardwood floor in our bedroom looking up at him and recalling what had happened only moments before.

"I was just walking across the floor, and I didn't slip, see?" I pointed to my feet since I didn't have any socks on. I had had a history of slipping on hardwood floors in my stocking feet in the past. "I was walking across the floor, and I felt lIke I was falling or spinning, and then I felt my head hit something." I made the assumption it was the door frame to the bedroom since my head was laying right next to it.

"Well, I never heard you scream so loud in your life." Dave said. He lifted me off the floor and helped put me to bed.

"That was scarier than shit. At least the last two other times I was sitting down," I said.

"Dave we have to do something. That was enough for me. Can you call Dr. Hain and see if he can get me in for an appointment? I need to know what the fuck is going on with me. It isn't right."

Calling Dr. Hain to get an appointment the day before was like asking the Pope to have coffee with you while you just happened to be visiting the Vatican. Normal appointments for one of the best Neurologists in the country are three months out so I wasn't too optimistic but we had to try.

After I slept for about three hours, my husband told me that we were in luck. There just happened to be a cancellation tomorrow at Dr. Hain's office. Someone was watching over my pathetic self.

My previous attacks were just as scary, but at least I didn't injure myself. The first one happened over the previous summer. I was sitting in my backyard enjoying the sun in my face when all of a sudden, I blacked out and thought I was falling forward and off to the side. I gripped onto the patio table and screamed for my husband. I kept asking him, "Did I fall over? DID YOU SEE ME FALL OVER??!" He kept telling me he hadn't, but it sure the hell felt like it.

A different time we had decided to walk into town for lunch. Sitting in the bar area, I started eating my sandwich, and I grabbed a hold of the table. "SHIT!" I said, and banged my hands against the table trying to hold onto something. Since we were friends with the bar owner, they allowed me to lay in one of the booths while my husband ran home to get the car and pick me up.

Embarrassing? Yes. Was there anything I could do about it? No. As my husband helped me out of the restaurant it was like watching someone escorting a drunk person out of the establishment, except no one kicked my ass to the curb. The drop attacks are different from my normal vertigo attacks. When drop attacks happen, there is no warning. The room just immediately spins and you feel like you're being picked up by something or someone and thrown across the room. They are scary because they happen out of nowhere. At least with the vertigo attacks I have some sense of them coming on - I don't have a lot of notice, but at least I can feel when they're approaching.

Whether I'm having a drop attack or a regular vertigo attack, I can pretend to be a mean drunk and start swearing at people, but all I want to do is lie down. Anyone can look and act like Otis from Mayberry if they really want to, but when you're not in the mood to poke fun at the situation - especially a situation that is spinning at rapid speed, Otis from Mayberry is the furthest thing from your mind.

Dr. Timothy Hain reminded me of Bill Gates. Similar in appearance and a very reserved personality, he sequestered us into one of his examining rooms and Dave and I explained to him what was going on. "You have what are called drop attacks, and this is very concerning to me," he said. Concerning to you??? You can imagine how I feel!

He went onto explain. "Drop attacks are the most severe form of Meniere's Disease. They typically occur without warning and are attributed to sudden mechanical deformation of the otolith organs (whatever those are), causing a sudden activation of vestibular reflexes. You suddenly feel like you are falling, although you are probably perfectly straight. It can certainly cause severe injury. Do you have stairs in the house?"

"Yeah. Does this mean I need to wear a helmet now?"

"Not a bad idea," he said. "But, we're going to try three different types of medical approaches to see if we can put a stop to the attacks."

Great. More meds. My liver will probably fail on me by the time I'm 50. I have a

bet with Dave that I'm on the seven year plan. Meaning that in seven years, I'll be

dead and gone and he won't have to nurse my sorry ass any longer. We have now

reduced the plan to two years. We were on the fast track.

The drop attacks were the most recent incident on the list of many incidents and

symptoms that I have had to deal with regarding Meniere's disease. My story

goes way back to when I was 21 years of age. I thought I was invincible. I had an

unquenchable taste for life and a constant overwhelming sense of staying ahead

of the pack. I wanted to be a leader.

Chapter 2 - I'm Invincible

I was young. I was partying like Madonna (this was back in the 80's). Dressing like "Material Girl," and going out to clubs with friends is what I did. 21 years old and loving my newly married life, hanging with friends. I had vigor and vitality!

It was around August. Don't expect me to remember the year, but if I did the math right (and I suck at math), it would take us back to 1985. My husband at the time and a few of our friends decided to go to the Kane County Fair. A yearly tradition in Illinois, the Kane County Fair is what you'd expect at any normal Midwestern county fair: Grilled corn on the cob slathered in butter, pig calling contests, rodeo shows, plenty of cowboys and carnival rides.

We decided to go on the Tilt-A-Whirl. For those who are familiar with carnival lingo, this fun little ride has you seated in a pod, so to speak, with about four or five other people. There's a big steering wheel in the middle, and the point is to make the pod swirl around on an unbalanced, turning, churning foundation and go as fast as possible.

I had never had a problem with any type of turning, swirling, upside-down type of ride in my life. I was the one who absolutely had to be seated in the very first car on the highest roller coaster in the world. I was the one who laughed when I would go face downward ten stories high and then loopity-loop it all over the damn park.

Not this time.

As the ride began to start, and my friends and I started to spin it faster and faster, I got sicker and sicker. My heart began to race so fast I thought I was going to have a heart attack. I started sweating. My face got numb. I began to scream, "STOP IT! STOP IT!" My friends knew something was terribly wrong, and the operator stopped the ride. I stumbled out, felt extremely dizzy and sick to my stomach.

After awhile I seemed ok. Maybe I was dehydrated. I mean it was August. We were drinking. I don't recall being drunk. I know I've done some stupid shit in my time, but I would definitely not get on a spinning ride while drunk.

Three months later I felt a fullness in my ears. It was the equivalent of talking in a large soup can....not that I had ever talked in or had a meaningful conversation within a large soup can before. I mean, who makes large soup cans for a person to fit into anyway? But, it felt like talking in a big, tin-like tunnel. My voice and everything around me sounded muffled. Scarcely audible, I had difficulty hearing

what people were saying around me. Initially I had thought it was sinus trouble.

But, after two weeks of dealing with it, I decided that it was more serious than

that. This is where I encountered my first visit with an ENT (Ear, Nose Throat)

Doctor.

I don't recall his name. Some Italian guy. Big nose and dressed like a pimp.

Cufflinks, tie clip (really? A tie clip?), and enough cologne to cause an evacuation

from "high cologne alert". Even back in the 1980's I thought tie clips were idiotic.

That's like a guy wearing a short sleeve shirt with a tie. You just don't do it. You

don't wear plastic pocket protectors either. My dad wore plastic pocket

protectors. But, in his defense it was the 1970's and he was an engineer. He was a

geek. He was allowed.

"You have Meniere's Disease," he said.

In a matter of fact tone I said, "Ok - so what do I take to get rid of it?" I sat on the

examining table swinging my legs back and forth and staring at his tie clip

thinking, "What's the reason for the tie clip, anyway? Are you a sloppy eater? Did you think it was going to be a bit breezy out today, so you had to tie down your tie with a tie clip?"

"We'll put you on a diuretic to bring the swelling down in the inner ear. But, you have to understand, that it may come back. If it does, make another appointment with me and we'll see if we need stronger medication."

At 21 years of age, you don't ask many questions of a doctor. I just kept thinking about his ridiculous tie clip. I didn't feel incredibly bad. I just had fullness in my ears at that time. No vertigo, no vomiting, no sleepiness or drop attacks. I grabbed the diuretics, heard some more "blah, blah, blahs" from the tie clip Italian pimp doctor and in about two week's time, my symptoms had disappeared. Did I look back? Hell no. I didn't even give a second thought to the doctor's comment about the fact that "it could come back."

I never considered that this particular incident at the young age of 21 would ultimately define who I am as a person at the age of 49.

Chapter 3 - Tinnitus Strikes

Anyone know what Tinnitus is? Raise your hand. Yes - you? No. It's not a musical instrument. No, it's also not a body part. Lastly, it is not a sexually transmitted disease. Tinnitus is that high pitched ringing in your ears. It. Just. Won't. Go. Away. EVER.

Tinnitus is commonly described as a ringing in the ears, but some people also hear it as a roaring, clicking, hissing or buzzing sound. It may be soft or loud, and it might affect both of your ears or only one. For some people, it's a minor annoyance. For others, it can interfere with sleep and grow to be a source of mental and emotional anguish.

My tinnitus is all of the above. High pitched ringing, roaring, or what some people call "loud bursts", clicking and buzzing. I don't get much hissing unless it's from a cat. I don't own a cat. However, the loud buzzing, clicking and roaring sounds were and still are, prominent in my ears 15 years later.

At first, it was extremely difficult to fall asleep listening to ten piece band playing in my head. But, after awhile I got used to the off tuned sounds and tried to actually make a game of it. Guessing what kind of song was playing in my head by the loud bursts and high pitched ringing, and also timing how long the loud bursts would last. Just for the record, they can last anywhere from a few minutes to a few hours. After awhile, they just kept on going. Tinnitus doesn't need batteries to keep them going. Your body will do that for you all on its own.

The one thing about loud bursts is that they are so loud, you don't even want to hear yourself talk. It's like hearing blood rushing thru your ears. It overwhelms your sense of hearing by blocking out just about everything else.

What I didn't understand at the time was how I got tinnitus. It wasn't until much later on thru my Meniere's journey I figured out that Meniere's disease was the underlying symptom of my tinnitus issues.

How I got Meniere's disease is still a mystery. Some people claim that it is caused by an ear infection that just never went away. If you recall in my earlier pages of this book, I had constant earaches as a kid. These earaches could have been a precursor to my Meniere's disease. So for parents out there with little kids take note: Forget the fucking ear drops. Get some strong antibiotics and definitely revisit the doctor to make sure the problem is gone!

Tinnitus started in my right ear. I was probably 35 at the time and just happened to wake up with it one day. It was one of those, "Oh, and by the way, here's some tinnitus for ya today." Again, thinking it was sinuses and not putting together the pieces that it may be Meniere's creeping up, I checked into some homeopathic methods of getting rid of it. I didn't realize that tinnitus can't be cured with a pill or any type of natural home remedy. So, I tried ear candles.

Why? Again, don't ask me that question because that was over 15 years ago. I think someone had told me about them and said that it really cleared up your hearing and could possibly help with the ringing in my ears.

It looks ridiculous when you try it, but ear candles really do clean out your ears. But, you need two people to handle the task or at least put yourself in front of a mirror so you can see the flame at the top of the candle. It's one thing to clean your ears of ear wax. It's another thing to clean your head of all your luxurious hair by having it get set on fire.

So, I laid my head on one side of the table and put the small end of the ear candle in my ear. My husband at the time lit the top of the candle with the lighter. The candles are made of linen and natural beeswax or sometimes other types of wax to help "collect" the stuff that comes out of your ear. It's like a funnel causing a tornado like effect in bringing up all the junk from deep within your ear that an average Q-tip can't reach.

After we had done one ear candle in each ear, I looked at what had come out and thought I could create a wax ear and submit it to Madame Tussad's House of Wax. That shit really came out of my ears? My head? What else is in there? A small child? Chopsticks? A hot wheel car?

The ear candles didn't work. I've also tried Gingo Biloba and Butcher's Broom. I know...Butcher's Broom? What the hell is *that* made of? All I can think of when I hear that name is an old Looney Tune show with Bugs Bunny and a witch who when leaving in a hurry left a flurry of bobby pins in her wake. She's the type of person who would use Butcher's Broom. I mean, she's a witch for Christ sake.

All of the holistic methods that I tried didn't work. My neurologist told me that holistic meds, especially for my condition, would do nothing to improve my health. Nothing did. As a matter of fact, shortly after I got tinnitus in my right ear, I had my second Meniere's attack. This time it was much, much worse. I was out of work for six weeks. I couldn't drive because I had terrible vertigo. I was vomiting from being nauseous, and just wanted to sleep all day. Sleeping all day as a parent is not an easy task. I was fortunate that my husband at the time had worked strange hours, so he was able to get our son ready for school in the mornings and take care of the basic needs a little boy needs.

As for me, the ENT doctor put me on a diuretic again and some anti-nausea medication. After six weeks I began to slowly feel better. The tinnitus remained and still does to this day. What I didn't realize at the time was that there was a much larger issue that I would not have even considered in a million years: I started to lose my hearing.

Gradual hearing loss is so subtle, you don't realize you are missing out on the little things. As an example, planes flying overhead weren't as loud. Birds chirping? I didn't notice they were there any longer. Leaves rustling in the wind or blowing along the ground during autumn were very faint, or almost non-existent. Typical house sounds that you're used to hearing: The furnace turning on, the dishwasher whirring thru its cycles, and certain creaks in the floor when you walk thru the house were no longer audible. I didn't notice this because these were small sounds I took for granted. It didn't affect my work. It didn't affect my relationships. They were just every day sounds that I couldn't hear any longer, and with my busy life I just didn't realize I no longer had the capacity to hear them.

I didn't notice.

Chapter 4 - What Was That? Pardon Me?

As you can imagine, gradual hearing loss will lead to more substantial hearing loss. In my mid to late thirties, I was starting to have trouble listening to people when they were whispering, or talking in a low voice. This often happened at work when my cube mate and I would talk about someone in the office or chat about the latest layoffs.

I started to ask "What did you say?" a lot. I didn't realize it until someone told me one day, "Are you having trouble hearing me? You keep asking me to repeat myself." It was only then that I had thought I may have a bigger issue other than tinnitus. And, remember - I wasn't aware that I couldn't hear birds any longer. I had taken these every day sounds for granted, so I didn't even realize I couldn't hear them.

When I got divorced and would go to clubs or bars where it was really noisy, I could hear people, but had to get close to the point of them yelling in my ear. Perhaps this was normal body language; getting into someone's personal space.

But, when you hardly knew them, it was not only uncomfortable for me, but I'm sure the other person felt kind of awkward as well.

I would go to the gym after work, turn my ipod up on high and run my 3 - 4 miles. Listening to music was great after working at the office. Running was even better. It was a great way to blow off some steam and not think about anything but my cadence and breathing. I would go home, and talk to Dave about our day, make dinner and watch some T.V.

The T.V. was always soft in volume. I would turn up the volume, and Dave would say, "Why is it so loud? Are you trying to break the sound barrier??"

"I couldn't even hear it. Is it that bad for you to listen to?"

With fingers plugged in his ears....."Yep."

Ok. Now, I knew I had an issue. Before the tinnitus wasn't affecting my work or personal relationships. But, now I was beginning to realize that maybe I had a hearing problem. If people kept asking me why I kept asking them to repeat themselves, and the T.V. was turned up to crack wall plaster, I was guessing it was starting to get on Dave's nerves as well.

"Honey, I think I should see an ENT about my hearing. Maybe I should check into those small hearing aids."

"I'm proud of you for admitting that," Dave said.

"Why? I mean, it's becoming a problem not only for me, but for you too. I'm surprised the dogs aren't covering their ears."

"No, I'm proud of you because it's a tough thing to admit. I'll go with you if you want."

At 41 years of age I needed hearing aids. Was it an easy pill to swallow? Well, to be perfectly honest I'm one of those people who, if I have a problem I just find a way to fix it. I mean, I don't want to keep having people repeating themselves, or driving my husband out of the house wearing earplugs. I'm a believer in Nike's tagline, "Just Do It."

So, I did it.

Have you ever been to an Audiologist? Sitting in a sound proof booth with ear phones and holding a button in your hand while raising your other hand to different tones, and listening to pre-recorded people talk either loud or soft into your head. It's fun.

Not.

Having me repeat words like, "hotdog, pirate, number, sasquatch, idiot, and porn star," was child like. Ok - they didn't have me repeat those *exact* words, but you get my point. And, after all of the testing, you look at the results. Circles with lines attaching to one another meant nothing to me. However, the Audiologist had pointed out to me that the audiogram showed that I definitely had some hearing loss in my right ear with not being able to hear high pitched or low pitched sounds. My left ear wasn't much better. I had hearing loss, but not as bad as the right ear.

"What is causing my hearing loss, do you know?" At this point, I was curious and concerned. The thought of wearing hearing aids was a life changer. Shit. I was listening to my ipod too loudly, wasn't I? It's all my fault. I KNEW IT.

"Do you have tinnitus?" she asked.

"Yes."

"Have you ever had Meningitis or severe migraines?"

"No, but I was diagnosed with Meniere's disease several years ago."

"Your hearing loss is most likely attributed to Meniere's." She went on to say that the tinnitus was the starting point of the hearing loss which just got more acute as time went on.

"So, what kind of hearing aids do I need? Please don't tell me I need the grandpa hearing aids. I can't really deal with that."

"No. You have to remember that hearing aids are used to amplify sound. Since your hearing loss is not a big issue at this point, we can fit you with hearing aids that can fit right into your ear. It will be subtle enough where people won't even see it, especially since you have long hair. Your hearing loss is not that bad. The "grandpa" hearing aids you're referring to, (the ones that wrap around the back of your ear), are for those people who have severe hearing loss. They are a more powerful hearing aid."

She took some string with a form snug for the ear and put it into my ear canal. She then filled it up with some sort of foam that solidified so it formed a mold for my ear. The string pulls out the mold when it hardens and it gets sent to their hearing aid people where it was custom fit for my ears.

With one battery compartment and a way to turn off and on the hearing aid with a little button in front, it was a very primal device and easy to use. The only issue was I had no control on how loud things could get. They made an "air hole" in the hearing aid so that air can circulate in the ear while the hearing aid was inserted. On a windy day, I felt like screaming, "Auntie Em! Uncle Henry! I want a cruller!"

They don't make crullers anymore. It's a shame, really. I think they're called donuts now.

Chapter 5 - The Old Radio

As my luck would have it, my hearing got worse. The hearing aids that fit so inconspicuously in my ears had to be replaced with the dreaded grandpa hearing aids.

I really hated these for a number of reasons. Now being 42 years old, I had to wear these large, heavy contraptions over my ears. You don't think they're that heavy when you hold them in your hand, but your ears certainly feel the strain after six or seven hours of wearing them. The other problem was that the rubber piece that fit deep into your ear had no way to provide air input, so my ears would get moist. This would cause itching. This would eventually lead to bleeding from the itching.

They were the most uncomfortable things I had ever worn and this includes Spanx. I don't even know why I tried Spanx. I mean, I didn't really need it. And, I'm one of those girls who doesn't like to sweat. But, I was given huge sweat glands by someone in my family and I have to use men's deodorant. This is not a joke. So trying to wear Spanx in the summer was no picnic. Let it all hang out, I say.

So, I'm living my life with my grandpa hearing aids and Spanx. What the fuck? Who needs to have trouble hearing and sweat at the same time?

Anyway, I digress.

In 2006, I decided to take some courses thru DeVry University in Web Graphic Design. The classes were designed for people with full time jobs, so they were developed as online courses. I started taking them in the fall when my dad was diagnosed with lung cancer.

I really loved the course work and it was something I had been dying to do for quite awhile. I had also been wanting to quit my Project Manager position I've held for so long, but the money was too good. However, this class offered me the opportunity to open up new doors and new challenges. Since they were online courses, I can do my work in the evenings or in between baseball and football games I attended for my son.

My dad died on January 3, 2007. I realized at that point I wanted to re-prioritize my life. I felt the need to make changes and do something "bigger."

So, I did what every normal woman would do. I got married.

In all seriousness, I was already engaged to Dave at that time. Thankfully, my dad was still alive when Dave had asked him the old fashioned way for my hand in marriage. With tears in his eyes, my father seemed grateful and thankful that I had found someone who was truly in love with me and would take great care of me. My father was right, because I was terrible at taking care of myself. Even though I worked out, I rarely took the time to eat right and was always on the go.

My father missed our nuptials on a cliff in Maui exactly one month later, but he was definitely there in spirit. It was just Dave and I since it was not a first marriage for either one of us. My mother was back home, as was my sister who was caring for her since my mom was ill with numerous health issues.

2007 was hard on our entire family. With the loss of my dad, my mom got sicker. Maybe it was from a broken heart, but she just seemed to give up on life. She also had undergone a personality change. She had become mean spirited and angry toward the people who were caring for her. As 2007 painfully wore on, my sister and I interviewed person after person to care for my mom because they were either fired by my mother, or they left due to my mother being too difficult to care for. My sister nor I did not have the experience to care for her. We also had full time jobs. Even though my employer was extremely understanding of my personal situation, I still felt guilty about leaving at a moment's notice, or had to take time off to take my mom to the doctor. But, as a daughter of an elderly parent, it was time to switch roles. My sister and I were now caring for my mother, as she had cared for us our entire lives.

It was stressful. We were still mourning the passing of our father. My hearing was getting worse. Exactly one year after my father's passing, my mother died on January 3, 2008.

With both parents gone within a year's time, I had done some hard thinking and talked it over with Dave. I was unhappy in my job. Enduring layoff after layoff and policy changes one after the other, I was fed up with the work environment. I would complain every night to my husband about what happened that day, and then it occurred to me:

What the fuck was I doing? I just lost both parents. Don't I have the insight to understand that life is short? If I'm so damn unhappy, then do something about it.

And, so I did.

I quit my job after ten years of being a Project Manager. I quit my six figure income to become a full time student and get my degree in Web Graphic Design. Why? Because it's what I *wanted* to do. I wanted the chance to have a shot at starting my own business.

Why the rush? To put it into perspective, when you lose both parents it became somewhat of an epiphany for me to change things - give myself a swift kick in the ass so I realize my time is limited; I was not immortal. I felt I had done all I could at my Project Management job and there was no room for growth. I had a creative side that was just trying to crawl out of my skin, and I wasn't able to utilize it there. So, I did what Nike told me to do. I just did it. Again.

During this entire time, my hearing became secondary to me. As you can imagine, there were larger issues to deal with. My sister and I had to go thru my parent's home and clear out everything. There were a lot of memories to sift thru, old photographs, clothes and jewelry. We threw out useless stuff, and then had an open house for our family to take what they wanted. Whatever was left, I sold in a garage sale and the proceeds were spent on dinner with my sister and her husband and Dave. Since my sister was the executor of the estate, she put the house up for sale just at a time when the real estate market started a steep decline. We were fortunate enough to sell it about seven months later.

It sounded so easy, didn't it? Emotionally and physically, my big sister and I worked side by side without a single argument. We were lucky in that respect. When parent's die, some kids will fight all the way to a judge's bench for a diamond ring. But, my sister and I were not brought up to be materialistic women. We were brought up to do the right thing. We loved each other. More importantly, we loved our parents and wanted to do right by them.

I retired from my Project Management position in March of 2008 and started going to school full time. The following month, I woke up one morning and felt "odd." That's the only way to describe it. I turned on the T.V. to check the weather for the day, and something became awfully strange and scary at the same time.

I couldn't understand what the weatherman was saying.

I could hear what he was saying since I had my grandpa hearing aids on, but I couldn't articulate the words. He sounded like gibberish. The best analogy I can provide is that he sounded like an old dial radio stuck in between stations. You could sort of understand what he was saying, but it was full of static. Incomprehensible.

I thought it was Meniere's again, but I wasn't dizzy. There wasn't any vertigo or nausea sinking in. The familiar feeling of fullness in my ears wasn't present. What was going on?

Dave was already downstairs, so I got out of bed and walked into the kitchen. I started a conversation with him and had the same result. I told him how I was hearing him, and the only way I could understand him at this point was by reading his lips.

And, so it started. My downward spiral into silence. I could hear, but not normally. Reading lips was my only salvation in addition to trying to listen to what people were saying thru my grandpa hearing aids. The other big problem since I woke up that April morning was that I could no longer hear on the telephone.

This whole situation had provided me a one way ticket on a secluded island. I was reduced to communicating thru my computer, texting, lip reading, hand puppets, pantomime and jazz hands. My ears didn't have a telephone touch them until well over a year later.

Coping with this newfound disability was not all it was cracked up to be. My "Just Do It" attitude was reduced to, "I don't know if I can do this anymore," attitude. The ability to hear like a normal person again was something I realized was no longer an option, and that scared the shit out of me. It frustrated my type A personality. It made me want to go ape-shit on someone because I just didn't get it. I mean, why me?

I had lost my sense of hearing.

Losing a sense taught me a few things. It allows your other senses to take over and compensate for the loss. To cope with not only not being able to hear properly, I had to come to the realization that I was missing out on a lot of conversations. To think about all of the meaningful topics and discussions people were having around me and all I could do was shake my head in agreement was extremely isolating and embarrassing. You can imagine conversations were difficult to hear, so when I would answer inappropriately to something it made me look like a complete idiot, unsympathetic, or I appeared as though I just didn't give a shit what people were saying to me. I started to look at people's body language to try to put pieces of information together and make a coherent storyline in my head about what certain discussions were about.

Hand gestures, facial expressions, body posture and positioning told a story for me. In noisy restaurants where I really couldn't hear anything, I would bring a small notebook and a pen. Dave and I would play a game. I would guess what the couple across from us was discussing, and Dave would tell me if I was right. 98% of the time I was correct. The notebook would get handed off between us hundreds of times over the next year, and we had a good laugh at some of the stuff we wrote.

If anyone had given you the choice of whether you wanted to be blind or deaf, I would choose being deaf any day. Being deaf allows me a degree of independence. There are some caveats to that: Communication is often an issue. If I didn't understand something, Dave would have to interpret for me. For instance, if we were in a restaurant and the waiter said something to me, Dave would interpret for me and say, "He said he wants you to leave because you're not wanted here." Or, "He says that he doesn't like you." The waiter would immediately look at Dave and say, "Ummmmmm No!" But, Dave was just like that....always. We poked fun at all the waiters. Most of them started calling us by name, and they would always...ALWAYS remember us when we came back into the restaurant. I wonder why....

Our home environment had to change. The TV didn't have to be loud anymore. Instead, we put on closed captioning. This was the worst situation for everyone involved.

Instead of me watching a television show, all I was doing was reading the lines scrolling across the bottom of the screen. Unfortunately, the closed captioning wasn't real time, so I was reading what had occurred on the TV screen about 15 seconds after it happened. The other problem were my poor husband and son. They had to endure the endless words moving across the screen. It would drive anyone insane if they weren't used to it.

To be honest, I never got used to it. Reading the TV made me tired and nauseous. The other problem is that I'm a huge grammar Nazi. The people who typed the closed captioning made me want to reach thru the TV screen and punch them in the throat. Horrible grammar and words spelled incorrectly made me not watch the TV very often!

I think the worst part waking up that April morning was that music was no longer an option for me. Hearing it either on the radio or thru my ipod just sounded like gibberish. Lady Gaga's "Poker Face" sounded like she was singing, "Cherry Pie." You can understand my frustration, can't you? I mean, why would she be singing about a dessert anyway? People had good laughs at my expense, but I laughed along with them because it *was* funny.

This was a big life changer. Not only for me, but for my family who had to live with me. You want to talk to me? Look directly at me. Don't talk to me while you're walking away because I won't be able to understand you. Want to watch a little TV? Do you mind watching and reading at the same time? Don't try to have a conversation with me while I'm upstairs and you're downstairs because it's pointless.

Theatres, concerts, plays, auditoriums of any sort were out. Outdoor festivals are fun for the gathering and wine drinking, but if you're there strictly for the entertainment, I was in for a huge disappointment.

Did you hear that huge thunderstorm roaring thru the neighborhood last night? Why, no. No I didn't. I was deafly sound asleep. What's that you say? My husband snores like a chainsaw? I didn't notice. What?! Burglar in the house? Wake me up so I can shoot his ass. I'm pretty good with a gun. Or, one of my German Shepherds will take him out. Or, shit! my husband can kill him with his bare hands.

I went back to the ENT Doctor. Diuretics again??? Please. I know the drill. After a week of being on them, the doctor indicated he really couldn't do much. Claiming it was Meniere's disease again, I simply would accept that as an answer. The symptoms this time were much different. I didn't have vertigo. I had a problem articulating speech in addition to my lack of hearing. I was told to see a hearing specialist at the Chicago Ear Institute - Dr. Battista.

Chapter 6 - Cochlear Devices

After seeing several ENT doctors, I was anxious to see this new guy, Dr. Battista. Will he walk in the examining room wearing shining armor and a vial of miracles so all this shit will go away?

Probably not. As my imagination was getting the best of me, I was meandering around the examining room. (Don't lie - you do it too): Washing my hands, drinking some water, looking at the spectacular view of the roof from the window, and looked at, but did not touch the several used and obviously finger licked pages of magazines in the wall holder.

I have a thing about used magazines. When you see a used magazine with pages that have been flipped thru time and again, they begin to curl. Why? Because people lick their fingers to flip thru the pages. Their saliva is on the pages. Therefore, my hands would probably be touching at least a hundred or so strangers' dried up saliva on those magazines. NO THANKS. I told this to a friend awhile back, and since then she thinks about it every time she looks at a magazine in a doctor's office or a hair salon. Think about that and get back to me.

But, one thing that caught my attention were some pamphlets sitting on one of the counters. On the front cover it read, "Are you a candidate for a cochlear device?" This is the first time I'd ever heard (no pun intended), about cochlear devices. It intrigued me. The image on the cover looked like a hearing aid, but it had a tether attached to it.

As I was reading the pamphlet is gave bullet points about people who would be a good candidate to receive a cochlear device:

Ask yourself the following questions. When wearing hearing aids do you:

- Experience difficulty hearing conversations, especially when there's background noise?

- Frequently ask people to repeat what they've said

- Misunderstand what people say

- Find it difficult to hear on the telephone

- Turn up the volume on the TV or radio louder than others in the room prefer

- Feel that people are mumbling or not speaking clearly when they talk

- Have difficulty hearing sounds of nature, such as birds chirping or rain falling

- Agree or nod your head during conversations when you're not sure what's been said

- Remove yourself from conversations because it's too difficult to hear

- Read lips to you can try to follow what people are saying

- Strain to hear or keep up with conversations

- Have trouble following the conversation when two or more people are talking at the same time

- Have a hard time keeping up with conversations at work

- Avoid social situations because you find yourself responding to the conversation incorrectly

- Experience tinnitus (a persistent ringing, buzzing or other sound)

If you answered yes to any of these situations, you may be a good candidate for a Freedom Nucleus Cochlear Device.

My heart stopped. I got anxious. This was me. It was a resounding yes to all of the above. I wanted more information, and just as I had finished reading the pamphlet, Dr. Battista entered the examining room.

As I handed him the pamphlet, I calmly said in three words, "I'm this person."

Dr. Battista was not a happy guy. I don't think I had ever seen him smile the entire time I had interacted with him. He was young and walked around with his laptop and lab coat while taking notes as we spoke about my situation.

He was very cognizant of talking directly at me and rounding his mouth perfectly to form words so I could read his lips easily. After a lengthy discussion which lasted about ten minutes, he wanted me to make an appointment with his audiologist to get tested to become a cochlear implant candidate.

When I left his office, I felt like I had a mission to complete. I had an option! I had a possible cure to my problems! There was hope!

For those of you who just read and then re-read those bullet points, you may see some similarities with what's happening to you.

What are Cochlear Devices?

Cochlear devices are a high tech way of hearing. Your natural ears just become ornaments to hold the devices in place and really serve no purpose physically since any hearing you did have prior to surgery would be "killed". It doesn't kill all the nerves in the ear, but it kills the nerves to your cochlear which is the central system for your body to have the capability to hear.

Being a two part process, they have to drill holes in your skull to place a steel plate (the size of a quarter) in the side of your head just above your ear. Then, they make an incision behind your ear, kill the cochlear organ you were naturally born with, and replace it with the high tech cochlear device.

The external device, or processor, which hangs on the backside of your ear has microphones and can be programmed for several different types of noise situations. These run on batteries that either can be rechargeable or disposable. Disposable batteries last about 5 days before they need to be replaced. Rechargeable batteries last about 12 hours before they take a dump on you mid sentence and you need to replace them. (As you can see, I'm a disposable battery gal). The sound gets amplified thru a tethered device with a magnet which gets attached to the steel plate in your skull, and those "waves" of information thru the sounds of the microphone get transmitted to your brain. Thus, your brain now has to re-train itself to certain sounds you haven't heard in awhile, or for people who were born deaf, the brain has to train itself on what these sounds are like.

I would be hearing thru my brain rather than my ears with this new form of technology.

The more I read about it, the more I wanted to have the surgery. I just needed to become a candidate so my health insurance would pay for it.

Chapter 7 - Candidacy and Insurance

When I first tested with the audiologist in Dr. Battista's office in July of 2008, my hearing loss was not significant enough to become a candidate for cochlear implants and have insurance pay for it.

There is one thing you need to understand about insurance: When people first started getting cochlear implants, insurance companies only paid for people who had profound hearing loss, meaning hardly any response to the loudest sounds. As the surgical techniques, implanted devices, and understanding of hearing with the implant had improved, these criteria had somewhat changed. Originally, most insurance companies made their decisions based on the audiogram - the hearing sensitivity report at different pitches. This is because of the original belief that only people with profound hearing loss should be implanted. Times started to change, however, and physicians and audiologists realized that people with more moderate losses in sensitivity and poor word understanding or clarity (as myself), could also benefit from the surgery. So word understanding is becoming the criteria for most insurance companies, rather than the audiogram. As far as word understanding goes, I was a good candidate for the device. However, my insurance company still used some of the old criteria. They saw my audiogram as borderline, and since my insurance company does not give pre-approval before surgery, they wouldn't guarantee whether or not I was a candidate by their standards. So, if I went ahead and had the surgery, my insurance company could deny the claim leaving me with a very large bill.

During 2008, cochlear surgery for each ear was $75,000.00. This did not include the devices which were $3,500.00 at that particular time and were NOT covered by insurance. Yeah.....Cha-Ching.

Without hearing and waiting for my hearing loss to get worse and re-test to see if I was a candidate, I felt helpless and at the mercy of my health insurance carrier. Talk about feeling like a prisoner! Talk about wanting to punch someone in the throat! My next re-test would have to wait until January of 2009.

I waited six long, isolating, frustrating months. January couldn't come fast enough. In the sound booth, we went thru the normal testing which typically takes about an hour to complete. Based on the audiogram it appeared I had suffered more than a 60% loss of hearing in both ears.

I was now a candidate for cochlear surgery. Finally.

When I spoke to Dr. Battista about the surgery he had explained that most people

get uni-lateral surgery (one ear at a time), and then come back in a few months to

a year to have the second surgery.

Not me. This "Just Do It," gal wanted both done at the same time. Bi-lateral

cochlear surgery isn't done very often simply because during post surgery the

person would be completely deaf for one month. This is a requirement in order

for the surgical incisions to heal before the devices are activated.

I didn't care about being completely deaf for one month. To me, I had been

completely deaf since April of 2008. I had had enough of this bullshit to last a

lifetime and wanted to improve the quality of my life. I wanted my hearing back.

I desperately wanted to be normal again.

Chapter 8 - Cochlear Surgery

Since April of 2008 and before then, I've had hearing issues. February 12, 2009 was the day that I had been anticipating for quite some time. I had never been put under anesthesia before. I had never had surgery before, but I wasn't nervous. I was anxious and feeling I was finally getting somewhere in trying to improve my quality of life.

As they readied me for surgery, they kept asking me my name, rank and serial number. The nurse was very kind and funny. No time for vanity here, folks. My gown wasn't made by Versace, although I really liked the non-slip socks they gave me.

Since this was a day surgery, I didn't need a hospital room, so I was kind of wondering how that whole post surgery thing worked. Do I have to just sit in the doctor's office and wait until my anesthesia wore off? Could I get a better outfit than this cotton drape? Do I get accessories? A purse, maybe?

They rolled me into the surgery room and I looked around. I had never been in one before and wanted to see what it was like. Nope. Not allowed. I saw lights above me, and a mask went over my face. "Begin counting backwards," someone said.

"100...99....80...."

When I woke up, I remembered nothing. I was reclining in something like a lazy-boy and I don't even know how I got there.

"You've been out for awhile," Dave said. "I was starting to worry they gave you too much anesthesia."

When he said that, I felt sick to my stomach. I needed to go to the bathroom, but I wasn't sure I could stand up straight. So, the nurse came in with a wheelchair and took me to the bathroom. As soon as I stood up after peeing, I fainted. She quickly gave me smelling salts which brought me back into the game, and they promptly put me back into the lazy boy recliner.

This is the part I didn't like. The nauseous feeling from the anesthesia was really getting to me. They gave me some crackers to settle my stomach, and Dave helped me get my clothes on so I wouldn't have to go home dressed in a cotton drape in February. The ride home was like a tilt-a-whirl. The bumps in the road just made me want to hurl into the windshield, but I held it together....barely.

Keep in mind, I had no idea what I looked like. At that point, I really didn't care. When I woke up the next morning and I had taken enough pain killers so that I was comfortable to see the damage, I asked for a mirror.

Two words: Princess Leia. My head was bandaged from side to side, and I had two huge "buns" on either side covering my ears. I had received two black eyes since the doctors and I got into a fist fight.

Kidding.

When they do the surgery, there is a lot of meandering the doctors' do thru nerves and muscles in your face. So, it looked like I was in the boxing ring and I let my opponent get the best of me.

I told Dave, "Well, this is attractive. Let's go to the store and have everyone look at my black eyes. I'll just point to you and say, "He did it.""

"Ok. Let me get my wife beater on."

"Awesome," I responded, even though I didn't understand what he had just said.

It took about two weeks for the black eyes to go away, but that didn't stop me from going out and running errands. People stared. People talked. Did I care? No. Did I listen? No. I was deaf.

From February 12 until March 11, 2009, I was completely deaf with no means to hear. Communication was done within my family using text messaging on the phone, hand puppets, lip reading, grandiose hand gestures and giving the middle finger.

My tinnitus was still evident (or maybe that was just my brain used to the sound for so many years). But, everything I did from the time I woke up until the time my head hit the pillow at night was done in silence. When I walked my dogs, I would have take a 360 view of cars and people before I crossed the street. People thought I was rude if I didn't respond to them if they made a comment to me. At times, I would get taps on the shoulder and people mouthing to me, "Did you hear me?"

That's the problem with being deaf. People can't *see* that you're deaf. It's obvious to a normal person when they see a blind person or someone who is handicapped. But, when you are a deaf person, you look normal. Shopping at the grocery store, I had no idea my cart was in someone's way until they would tap me on the shoulder with a surly look on their face. I often apologized for my inadequate means to hear. And, I think that when I responded in perfect language that "I am deaf," they probably didn't believe me because there is a stigma in America that deaf people can't talk right. I can. I just talked loud - and still do.

I anxiously awaited activation day and couldn't wait to be able to hear again.

Chapter 9 - Activation Day

Long expected and highly anticipated, the turning on my cochlear implants came on March 11, 2009.

Walking into the audiologist's office was like Christmas morning. She handed me two big yellow boxes.

Each one was equipped with accessories and my cochlear device for each ear. I didn't anticipate so much "equipment." Each box contained more boxes. They were appropriately labeled: Accessories, documents and batteries. There was also a dehumidifier.

Yes, a dehumidifier. The dehumidifier was to be used to take out the moisture from your cochlear device at the end of each day to keep it in proper working order.

The accessories ranged, among other things: Monitor earphones, extra battery compartments, ear hooks, extra control panels and various cables.

After we went thru the contents of each box and she showed me the cochlear

devices, she showed me how to put the batteries in. She then asked me to put

them around my ears and attach the tether to my head.

A cord was connected to her computer to my cochlear device. I hung the device

on my right ear first and connected the tether magnet to my head.

Then I heard her. "Can you hear me?"

I heard her. She sounded like she was from the Emerald City. Dave, the

audiologist and myself all sounded like munchkins. From a technical standpoint,

your brain is now doing the hearing for you, so I had to put my brain through

some personal training sessions on how to re-learn sounds that were once

familiar to me: My voice, my husband's voice, normal house sounds, dogs barking,

crinkling of paper, water running...you name it.

The audiologist had explained to us that upon initial activation, it was completely

normal for people to hear others' sound like they were non-humans, or robots. If

you worked at re-training your brain to hear what you used to hear, odds were

pretty good that the old familiar sounds you loved and cherished would come

back. However, there are some people who aren't so lucky, and the familiar voices and sounds that they would typically recognize would no longer be an option for them. Why? Maybe it's age. Maybe it's because they were born deaf to begin with. Maybe it's because they've been hard of hearing for so long that their brain has truly forgotten what the chirps of a bird are supposed to sound like.

When we walked outside after our visit with both cochlear devices firmly in place, I stopped and listened.

"Dave, what's that noise?"

He said, "Those are birds chirping, honey." I realized the sounds I had taken for granted like birds chirping or leaves rustling thru the wind were not sounds I had heard in probably five years.

I cried.

Not because I was able to hear these simple sounds again, but because I realized how much I had missed in my life all those years due to my progressive hearing loss. It was unfathomable. Five years is a long time to miss out on normal stuff you should have been able to hear. Was I angry? Yes. Was I sad? Yes. Did I have a pity party for myself? Yes. Did I get over it? Eventually. Please read on.

I could hear again. I look at it this way: Look forward and don't look back.

For six weeks, I would go back each week to see my audiologist and get a "fine tuning." The processors have different programs: One is for normal hearing environments, like your home. A second program can be used for the phone, and a third setting can be used for louder situations like restaurants. There was volume control and circumference mode to maintain how far out you wanted to hear things. We tweaked the sounds and pitches until it was comfortable for me to live with on all levels.

Whether I'm walking my dogs or doing yard work, I don't listen to music. I listen to nature. I listen to trucks roaring by. I listen to my voice yelling at my dogs for trying to chase the UPS trucks. It's amazing how much you miss the simple sounds in life.

It's also kind of frightening listening to your voice thru your brain. This one is really hard to explain, but if you have normal hearing, you can always hear yourself talk, but when you hear yourself on an answering machine, or a video, you always think you sound different than what your voice truly sounds like. With me, there is no difference. Since I hear thru my brain I hear my voice thru technology already. Hearing myself in a video or on a voicemail makes no difference to me. I sound exactly the same.

When I would sleep at night, it would seem to me that I would be picking up radio stations. It was alarming at first because the music playing in my head was the exact replica of the Bee Gee's, "Stayin' Alive," or Tony Orlando and Dawn's famous song, "Knock Three Times." I swear.....*SWEAR,* these songs were coming from a satellite dish from up in space. The steel plates in my head were sending me signals. The songs were just like listening to the radio all over again. The detail of the songs was spectacular.

It was not to be. My audiologist explained to me that it was common for the brain to play "tricks" on you and recall certain sounds and even songs to retrain itself. My brain took it upon itself to go into juke box mode and randomly select songs it thought I would remember specifically for my entertainment. What a true, fine and genuine brain I had. Although I'm thankful for my brain for keeping me entertained during the early morning hours, it picked the wrong time to play with me because I WANTED TO SLEEP.

Chapter 10 - The New Normal

It took about a month for my brain to catch up and then it decided it didn't like what was happening.

I started to have vertigo. This is the room spinning, body twirling thrill ride that happens inside your head while you sit perfectly still.

Still unable to use the phone, Dave called Dr. Battista and we went in for an appointment. "You're encountering positional vertigo. It's a common side effect from cochlear surgery, so you'll need some rehabilitation to train your brain to re-balance itself."

My brain needs rehab? What about my juke box? Please don't show me any Rorschach patterns or make me play the memory game, or put a square peg into a round hole. I'm thinking big flash cards, like the ones in grade school. And, Twister is definitely not an option. I know my colors, thank you very much.

In all honestly, the rehab was kind of fun. The therapist who helped me gave me a bunch of exercises to do each week. One of them was having Dave throw a tennis ball to me from behind, where I would have to catch it by looking side to side and back at him in order to catch the ball. We did this while walking down our street every night. I'm sure people who saw this in our neighborhood were thinking we were fine tuning our circus act, because throwing knives of fire at one another just wasn't conducive to our otherwise perfect relationship. Insurance costs were skyrocketing. You know how it is.

About a month later, the ball throwing, reading big print while moving my head side to side, and other exercises seemed to have helped. I had also come to the sad realization that there are just some things that cochlear devices can't replicate as well as I had hoped when it comes to natural hearing. One of them was music, and I was stuck like Aqua Net in the big hair of the 1980's.

With the wonders of technology and the big yellow box I received on my activation day, there were cords that I could connect via a splitter to my iPod. The only way for me to be able to understand music was thru my iPod. The list of music that I could understand was limited to what I listened to as a kid and had heard prior to surgery. It was music my brain recognized so it didn't take long to catch onto the tune. It was like the juke box in my head I mentioned earlier.

Post surgical songs sounded meaningless. I couldn't understand them either on the radio or thru my iPod. It would take about eight times of listening to the same song on my iPod to finally get the beat of the song and barely understand the lyrics like Lady Gaga's, "Cherry Pie." (Poker Face).

After six months of feeling pretty good, I started having headaches. Not bad ones, but headaches that would make me feel a little "off." Kind of dizzy, but enough to still function. It felt like that saying, "I got up on the wrong side of the bed this morning." As the months went on, the headaches got worse. One day, as I was working on the computer, I had a deadly spin.

I stopped typing, took off my glasses and grabbed my head. "Holy shit," was all I could say. I couldn't see straight. My eyes felt like they were darting back and forth at a rapid pace. I immediately felt sick to my stomach. As luck would have it, I was on the second floor of my home, so I was able to crawl from my office to my bedroom. I tried to stand up, but couldn't even try to balance myself - my body had taken over the thrill ride controls and it was well, out of control. I managed to crawl into the bed and close my eyes to let the vertigo pass.

It took six hours with a bucket by my side.

A few days later, it happened again. This round lasted eight hours. How was I supposed to function like a normal person? When these episodes happened, my husband was right there to help me, thank God. And, one day while out running errands with my son, I had an episode in an art store which required him to escort me to the car - kind of like Sheriff Taylor escorting Otis to his cell, and have him drive me home, and he was only ten.

I'm kidding.

He was seventeen at the time with a valid driver's license. I don't know what I would have done without either of them throughout this entire journey.

Most of 2010 was spent in vertigo hell. Doctor visits thru two Neurologists, numerous medications, constantly sick, I was spending more time sleeping than I was awake. I finally came across a third, brilliant Neurologist that my current doctor at the time had recommended.

Dr. Timothy Hain is a widely recognized leader in the field of otoneurology. He is a Professor of Neurology, Otolaryngology and Physical Therapy at Northwestern University. I was also impressed that he is among Chicago's Top Doctors for otoneurology, dizziness and motion sickness.

It took me three months to get an appointment with him, but it was worth the wait.

The initial impressions and final diagnosis:

1. Bilateral Meniere's disease

2. Migraines without headache.

So, basically what's happening is that because I have bi-lateral Meniere's disease, I'm twice as lucky. The loud attacks from my tinnitus is also twice the fun. So, if I get to have twice the fun because I'm twice as lucky, I get to have not twice, three or four times the Vertigo episodes, but by gosh! I'm a big winner here! I get to have hundreds of them!

After a year of being so sick, I had finally had a solid diagnosis. However, it came at a psychological price.

Chapter 11 - Dizzy and Depressed

As you can imagine, since my cochlear surgery in 2009 I had been pretty ill most of 2010 since that's when my issues got serious.

On top of losing my ability to hear, I had also lost both of my parents within a year. I retired from my job to embark on a new career and I had a new marriage.

I consider myself a happy person. You can normally see me doing the silly stuff that people would never do in public, being the opinionated one, I always have something to say. But, in 2010 it took me awhile to realize or maybe I just didn't want to realize it that I was suffering from depression.

The tipping point to this was when I would wake up in the morning I would cry. My eyes barely open from a previous night's sleep, I would slowly wake up and dread going thru another day. It all felt so meaningless. I mean, me. I felt meaningless. Plus, the two most influential people who could help me thru this ordeal with their constant encouragement were dead.

I was just plain sad. I would get anxious whenever I had to use the phone. I couldn't sleep. I had thoughts of dreaming that if I died, I would feel relief and pleasure because I would be able to hear naturally again. I wouldn't have to deal with all the sickness or feeling left out of conversations because I couldn't understand anything. I was sick of wearing hardware on my head. If I sweat, they would automatically turn off. Batteries would go dead while I was talking mid-sentence. They were heavy.

I wanted my hearing back. I lost being me.

I missed being me and felt there was no way to get myself back.

What was even worse than losing myself, was the fact that I had a husband who had bought into this relationship. He endured the death of my father one month before we got married, he dealt with the death of my mother and now my hearing loss and all my issues that went along with it. I felt extremely saddened and guilty to have put him thru these trials and tribulations. You see, my husband is my rock. He's fought in numerous wars during his almost 30 year tenure in the army.

My husband deserved some peace and tranquility in his life. I failed in that respect. The guilt I carry on my shoulders for burdening him with my illness is not something I take lightly. Married couples should vow to love one another in "sickness and in health" among other things. But, in my opinion, my husband deserved better than what I had to give him. I didn't feel worthy of his love because I was sick all the time. I guess I just didn't feel like it was fair to him. He didn't sign up for this. But, then again - neither did I.

I didn't care about anything except the fact that I was feeling a profound sense of loss and knowing that I would never get my hearing or my mom and dad back. It was just too much loss within a short period of time, and the feeling of depression - the feeling of loss had finally caught up with me. I told Dave that I thought I needed to see someone. I felt that something was truly wrong with me. After I told him everything, I received a name of a great therapist thru a friend I had known for twenty years.

When I entered the therapist's office, and I didn't even know what to say. Having never been in this type of situation, I felt speechless and nervous. I know - me speechless. But, there I was feeling ready to bare my entire life to this stranger and I really wasn't very comfortable with it. I was anxious, nervous and extremely sad. The therapist who worked with me was kind and earthy. She was a great talker, and helped to open up the conversation. Her office smelled like incense with a lot of artifacts from Africa placed around the room. After she spoke about herself for awhile, she then asked me why I was there to pay her a visit. It was then that the flood gates decided to open and the water from the tears I shed became a sea unto which I wasn't sure I would be able to sail on.

It was tough. I don't open up to people easily. We covered plenty of ground from my childhood all the way up until the reason why I walked thru her door. I won't go into details about the sessions. I don't want to.

It took about six months to get me back on the right track. I realized that my current situation - my life as it is now - is my new normal. This is who I am. I had to learn how to worry more about how I felt and less about what people might think. Letting go of those negative feelings and setting new boundaries was my mission.

My therapist gave me some guidelines on who to stay away from. If a person hears my story and actually feels shame for me by saying, "I'm so sorry," it's often followed by an awkward silence and I then need to make *them* feel better by telling them, "It's not your fault." Actually, this happens all the time. I don't know whether people say those three words because they just don't know what else to say, or it's just a knee jerk reaction to a horrible story. I find myself doing the same thing to be quite honest.

A few other people who should stay out of my personal space:

- The person who needs me to be the pillar of strength. They hear my story and all of a sudden I'm a big disappointment. It makes me feel like someone auditioning for the musical, "Annie."

"The sun with come out tomorrow - bet you're..."

"Thank you. We'll call you. NEEEEXXXT!"

This so called friend now wants nothing to do with you. So much for friends.

- The friend who likes to one-up you. You know the one: "Oh, you think your situation is bad, let me tell you about my Aunt Bethany."

- The friend who says, "Oh, I know exactly how you feel." Really? You're deaf too? You have spinning migraines and fall at the drop of a hat? Let me tell you how I feel about that by expressing it in sign language. You know how to sign "the bird," don't you, because that's the only damn sign language I know.

- The friend who says, "Aw, c'mon! it's not that bad! I'm sure you're just exaggerating. You're a rock! You can go thru anything!" To that person, all I can say is that you have never seen my reaction to seeing a spider on the wall.

- The person who says, "You're so brave for dealing with this." This is what the definition of bravery is to me: Putting your life on the line. Simple, isn't it? The term that is more applicable here is being vulnerable, not brave. Not having a choice in putting my vulnerability out there is a better definition.

I understand that people really mean no harm when they say things like this. But, when you hear it over and over again, it just makes me want to punch them in the throat. They don't know what it's like. They can't compare me to someone else, and I don't need their fucking pity. What I want is to be normal before all this shit happened. I want to go to loud restaurants and still be able to hear people. I want to listen to music without having to repeat it over and over and over again. I don't want to keep telling people that I'm a little hard of hearing. I want to be able to have a normal conversation on the phone and not worry about the inability to hear the person on the other end.

Since all of this was now a distant memory, I had to settle for my new normal.

At this point, I was able to use the phone, but the phone didn't quite like my devices. Or, maybe it was my brain that just didn't like the entire combination. Talking on the phone was a real struggle. Dave and I eventually did some research on the best phones to use for cochlear devices, or any type of device that has T1 coil capability, and purchased the best one we could find. It definitely helped. I still have problems at times, but it's much better than it used to be. Just don't hook me up with some guy from a helpdesk line in India.

As I'm getting used to my cochlear devices, it certainly didn't stop my vertigo issues. Between 2010 and now I've gone thru countless attacks. I'll never the forget the time I was working on my computer and I had a spin attack. This time, I couldn't even get to the bedroom. I felt so sick, I crawled to the bathroom and threw up. Thankfully, I didn't miss the toilet. Out of the three that I saw, I picked the middle one and lucked out.

I was smart enough to have my phone on me, but I had one problem: My eyes were darting back and forth too quickly, so I couldn't read or even see clearly the numbers. So I laid on the bathroom floor and covered myself with one of the floor mats. I was alone at home. My son came home three hours later.

I could feel the thumping of someone walking up the stairs, so I started knocking on the bathroom wall. I kept knocking rather than yelling, because I couldn't hear anything since I took out my devices to try to calm my vertigo. My son finally located me and I handed him my cell phone.

"Call Dr. Hain for me, and hand me the phone."

Matt called the number and explained to the nurse who I was and how I was casually lying on the cold, ceramic bathroom floor with a floor mat over my body. He gave me the phone.

"I'd like to consult with Dr. Hain on my medications. They aren't helping me any longer."

I've had vertigo attacks in my living room, kitchen, countless restaurants, and one at my hair salon. I had a drop attack while I was getting my hair dyed. Picture me with a black plastic drape buttoned around my neck and my hair all full of hair dye. I'm sitting there, not feeling so good. To be honest, I thought that maybe I should cancel my appointment, but shit - getting my hair done and having a facial were the two things I really looked forward to in life, so I wanted to treat myself, and nothing was going to stop me, damnit!

Sitting there in the salon chair, I wasn't able to read, so I just was looking at people's lips and trying to understand conversations. (since I was getting my hair dyed, I wasn't wearing my cochlear devices). Then it happened. A nice speedy spin. I grabbed onto the counter and apparently screamed. A few girls came rushing over and not being able to hear them, or myself for that matter, I told them what was happening and to call my husband to pick me up.

Then I realized the horror: I still had hair dye in my hair. Fuck. FUCK! Now, I have to lay my head back and get it rinsed off?!! A spinning head and lying backwards into a sink. You can imagine how that felt. Well, you probably can't, but it sucked. I started crying. I knew crying did absolutely nothing for my condition so I was mentally trying to calm myself down.

The salon allowed me to lay down in one of their massage rooms until Dave came and picked me up. With my wet curly hair dangling over my face, I barely made it into the car. We drove home and I slept for four hours.

My husband can always tell when I'm about ready to have a vertigo attack. He can read my eyes. They appear to dart back and forth before I actually have an attack. My head feels cloudy and I slowly have that spinning sensation.

Drop attacks are different. No warning. No signs. It just feels like I'm being picked up by some demon and thrown across the room, when in fact, I'm sitting (or standing) perfectly still.

Chapter 13 - Finding the Right Cocktail

Trying to find the right medicine to work with your body is like going to a crowded bar with a litany of martini choices. Which martini is the best for your taste buds?? I don't advocate mixing alcohol with medication, but that's the only analogy I can come up with right now.

Since September of 2010, I have experimented with the following medications:

- Nortriptyline - This was a typical medication subscribed by doctors to reduce migraines. It's also an anti-depressant. For some reason, anti-depressants act as a deterrent to the effects of migraines.

- Topiramate - Topamax (topiramate) is a seizure medication, also called an anticonvulsant. It can be used alone or in combination with other medications to treat seizures in adults and children who are at least 2 years old. It's also used to prevent migraine headaches in adults. It will only prevent migraine headaches or reduce the number of attacks. It will not treat a headache that has already begun. It rare cases, it also causes depression and thoughts of suicide. (Yeah, this was a bad mistake).

- Propranolol - is a beta-blocker. Beta-blockers affect the heart and circulation (blood flow through arteries and veins). It's used to treat tremors, angina (chest pain), hypertension (high blood pressure), heart rhythm disorders, and other heart or circulatory conditions. It is also used to treat or prevent heart attack, and to reduce the severity and frequency of migraine headaches.

None of these worked. You also have to understand that I had been on valium (2mg) since 2009 in order to help treat the vertigo which helps to a degree.

Some medications gave me low blood pressure. Every time I would stand up, I would feel like fainting. Other medications made me depressed (go figure). And, others made me lose my appetite. The last problem wouldn't be so bad if you truly wanted to lose some weight, but I was already slim. Dropping 30 pounds made me buy some new clothes. Perk? Possibly. But, I would rather drop the 30 pounds thru another method!

This is what I'm currently taking:

- Venlaflaxine - is used as an anti-depressant to treat major depressive disorder (MDD). Again, anti-depressants have a compound related to assisting in the reduction of migraines.

- Diazepam - Valium, as we all like to call it, is what I've been steadily taking with 2 mg tablets 4 times a day. Yes, I am addicted.

- Betahistine - This medication is used to treat dizziness (vertigo) in those who have Meniere's disease. I take this tablet four times a day along with the valium.

- Verapamil - This is in a group of drugs called calcium channel blockers. It works by relaxing the muscles of your heart and blood vessels. It's used to treat hypertension, and blood flow. I take one pill a day.

- Divalproex - This medication is used to treat seizure disorders, certain psychiatric conditions (manic phase of bipolar disorder), and to prevent migraine headaches. It works by restoring the balance of certain natural substances (neurotransmitters) in the brain. I take one pill a day. If I took anymore than what was prescribed, I'd start losing my hair and I wasn't too cool with that.

So, you'd think I would be pretty relaxed with taking all these meds. Most people would say, "I'd be a zombie most of the day." My body is so used to taking the meds I'm on, I'm really ok with all of it. Any side effects are met with a "well, ok" kind of attitude. This is my new normal, remember?

I simply do a comparison of the quality of life I had lived between 2010 and today, and right now....at this very moment I'm feeling pretty good and I'm grateful for that.

I was recently put on the Betahistine and Verapamil due to the drop attacks I was having which started in August of 2012. So far, as of this writing, I haven't had a problem for over a month - at least with the drop attacks. But, as I'm well aware of this disease, it progresses. I'm desperately hoping it doesn't go any further than this.

Chapter 14 - Limitations

I can say that being a type A personality, there should be no limitations in doing what you want to do. However, I think the hardest thing I've had to encounter is the fact that I DO have restrictions on what I can and cannot do.

Have you ever given consideration to what it would be like to be deaf. Not hearing a single sound. Sure, it's quiet in your house, but you still hear sounds. I would like to think the sensation would be equitable to being underwater, but that would not be a true statement. You can still hear things while being underwater: waves swishing and people talking above the water yelling or laughing. Deafness is pure silence. When something big drops to the floor, I "feel" the thump it made. When my dogs bark, I can't hear them, but if they jump on my bed while I'm sleeping, I can feel they are present to wake me for a incoming visitor, burglar, tornado or other natural disaster.

My everyday life is vastly different from yours. I wake up deaf. I shower without sound and get ready for my day without any noise. I don't wear my cochlear devices immediately upon awakening, because it spurs vertigo attacks. My brain needs to have a chance to rise and greet and day as well. Once my devices are put on my head, I consider my day officially started.

- Did I miss a call?

- Check my email.

- Did I receive a text message from my husband or my son?

- Was there a package delivered?

- Do the dogs need to go outside?

These are things I check because I may have missed the sounds to alert me that I needed to take action.

There are limitations to my day to day activities. I can't go to concerts or large outdoor settings with music or lectures because I wouldn't understand what they were saying. I certainly don't want to keep burdening my husband with my constant, "what did he say?" questions. I also have to avoid noisy places. Bars at 10 pm at night or a room with a lot of people bring about my loud bursts which change into migraines and quickly make me go into spin mode.

I avoid negative people. Some have called me a liability. I once had a part time job and was helping a customer. She was a "low talker," so I took out my remote for my cochlear device to turn up the volume. She stepped back with an alarmed look on her face at what I was doing. I explained to her what it was used for. She then asked if knew sign language and started signing with her hands. I explained that I didn't understand sign language. She gave me an angry look and said, "You're full of shit!" She didn't believe I couldn't hear because I didn't understand sign language. What's the sense of using sign language when the rest of your family doesn't understand it?

I think there's a social stigma between people who are absolutely deaf with no alternative and can't use cochlear implants, compared to those who can. It's like Republicans and Democrats. People who can't get cochlear implants use sign language. Cochlear implant recipients don't need to understand sign language because they can hear thru their brain. Yet, the people who only use sign language see cochlear recipients as people who have left their group - they are now traitors and using a different form of communication.

I don't listen to music any longer. I will listen to Christmas music because it makes me happy and I recognize it right away. I will listen to my iTunes choices if I'm working on my designs, but it's really just used as background noise. I don't get up and dance like I used to. My husband is happy about that.

I often hear odd sounds and wonder where it's coming from. Dave will tell me, or the dogs will let me know what's going on.

Balance is an issue. I am now a clumsy oaf. I've fallen down stairs, slipped on floors, and banged into door frames. It takes me longer than I used to in order to complete certain tasks. This is simply because I just can't have my eyes dart back and forth along with my head moving side to side without some kind of ill side effect.

Getting a permanent in your hair is also no longer an option if you have cochlear devices. Why? The chemicals for a hair permanent do not adhere or affect hair that has metal underneath it. I figured this out after two attempts at getting a loose wave in my hair. The first time I had it done, I called up my hair stylist and told her that the sides of my hair looked limp, and not curly like the top and back of my head. So, I went back into the salon and tried a different type of perm. The same thing happened. I looked like I poodle with a Mohawk for six months.

Did I set a new trend in hair styles? I think not. Vogue and In Style magazine weren't busting down my door for cover shoots, so I guess my perm was a big, fat, semi-curly bust.

At times I still feel secluded and unaware of conversations, music, and things that have happened around me which I wasn't aware. I don't complain because this was handed to me by someone much more powerful than I. This was given to me for a reason. I think about these reasons often and the few that mostly pop into my head are:

- All of these things were handed to me so that I was forced to slow down and not go ape shit at a moment's notice. Being on valium, anti-depressants and anti-seizure medication has its benefits. My son is lucky he's still alive.

- Since my pace in life has slowed down, so has my reactions. Physically and mentally. It causes me to think before I act.

- Having this disease - the journey into which I didn't want an invitation, gave me the opportunity to educate and help others' who have the same problem.

My situation is unique. Most people that I talk to are either just deaf in one ear, or have problems hearing. Some speak about a relative who refuses to recognize the fact that they have a hearing issue. If you are one of those people who knows you have hearing loss and are reading this book, please get yourself to an ENT specialist who can diagnose your situation and make life easier not only for yourself, but for the people who love you. You have no idea what you're missing out on in life.

I am a realist. I believe and see the signs ahead of me to take action. At times, I regret having cochlear device surgery in both ears since I don't even use my left device any longer to help reduce the amount of meniere's attacks I receive. But, I live with my choices and can't go back.

You can't reverse hearing loss. You can't get back all of the moments in time that you missed important conversations and events. Am I bitter for it? No. What good would it do? I would rather live my life with what god has handed me in the best way I know possible and avoid negativity.

Negative feelings make people look old. I don't need any more wrinkles. I'll take laugh lines though!

Chapter 15 - Resources

The Cochlear website is a great source of information about types of devices, candidacy, forms, costs, etc.

Chicago Dizziness and Hearing is the website for Dr. Timothy Hain.

Chicago Ear Institute is the place to get tested for candidacy and meet the surgeon who would perform your cochlear surgery.

Dehumidifier Packs website. Since you need to replace the drybricks in your dehumidifier, you'll need to know where to get them.

Not sure you're a Meniere's patient? Check out this flowchart thru Chicago Dizziness and Hearing.

Do you have tinnitus? Read this flowchart to see if you've gone thru all the steps necessary to help resolve the problem.

Made in the USA
Lexington, KY
21 June 2013